HOW TO GROW YOUR PENIS
Techniques To Naturally Increase the Size of Your Penis

Introduction

I want to thank you and congratulate you for downloading the book, *"How To Grow Your Penis"*.

This book has lots of actionable techniques on how to naturally increase the size and girth of your penis with no equipment.

This might sound unpleasant but it's a fact: We are living in a masculine world. We are living in a world that is idolizing masculine values- even our own language indirectly conveys this fact. Many words and expressions such as "man up" that mean "be strong/brave" assert (though indirectly) how the world views masculinity.

Among other issues such as general body physique, you'll find that most men actually care so much about improving sexual performance- they want to have longer sex and protect their masculine image in this respect and if they think the penis size is the deterrent, it can lead to stress and anxiety if there is no available, working solution. I believe this is only a natural response to the expectations of the world we live in and the societal demands we cannot escape from.

Think about it; most women wouldn't want to give you any hope of having sex with you if they think you are not just 'gifted' down there. If you have a small penis, perhaps showering with men around you will constantly remind you of how lacking you are in that area of your life irrespective of how successful you are in other spheres of life. Obviously, your ego will be constantly bruised when the topic of penis sizes, sex and related topics come up. And even when you go to urinals and other men who are 'gifted' well don't shy from holding theirs with pride for anyone who cares to look to see it, you will constantly feel bad about yourself and how lacking you are. Your self-confidence and self-esteem takes a nosedive, which subsequently affects other aspects of your life.

If you are tired of being shy about your small penis and perhaps have experienced any of the problems above, let this book be the beginning of the end of your silent suffering. With this book, I'll be focusing on the 'member'. Do you have doubts about your penis size? If your answer is a sorry 'yes', don't worry; I will teach you how you make your penis larger (in girth and length) to change how you feel and think about yourself completely for the better, the natural way i.e. no tools/equipment needed!

Thanks again for downloading this book. I hope you enjoy it!

About The Author
Daniel D'Apollonio

Daniel is a publisher of written content and online books from Adelaide, South Australia. His passion for philanthropy has led him towards people and travel, and when not giving back he can be found focusing on his own self improvement.

Daniel publishes books within various genres, and all can be found online. All of the content that Daniel provides is unique and engaging, offering relevant advice regarding a variety of topics of common interest.

If you love Daniel's picks, take advantage of his other free publications, today. Recent published works include, "Juicing For Beginners: Secrets To The Healthy Benefits Of Juicing", and, "Bodybuilding: Building The Perfect Body With Simple Hints And Tips That Will Give You Dramatic Results".

Daniel offers all of his publications free of charge for public enjoyment. Join his list of people and get updates when new *free* titles come into the market, and dont forget to look at his authors page for his already *free* titles! Enjoy!

Click here to get Notified of Daniel's Free releases

And

Click here to check out Daniel's Free titles on his Authors account

Table of Contents

Before we start with the specifics of how to grow your penis naturally, let's start by understanding the nasty experiences/consequences of having a small member. Perhaps if you associate with any of these consequences, you may feel compelled to do something about your member.

The Nightmare Of Having A Small Penis

✓ **Reduced Self-Confidence/Self-Esteem**

The most obvious effect of having a small penis is lack of self-confidence. Many men believe that having a bigger member means being able to perform really better sexually and having stamina. Your lack of confidence can be depicted in many areas, such as during casual friends' chat whereby you deviate from the sex talk or any other that involves the use of the penis. Your ego becomes completely washed up once others begin observe that your penis will never be 'used well'. Sometimes it gets worse- the self-esteem becomes so damaged that you may even decide to not have sex at all (many have confessed that they are still virgins at 50 due to lack of confidence). And the society makes this problem worse:
The reinforcements around you
As a man suffering from this 'small penis syndrome', you'll find that you are always bombarded with visual and verbal reminders that you don't measure up.

You are reminded that having a small penis means that you are extremely inadequate in all other facets in life and not just sex. You will meet average size or large sized men in public showers, locker rooms, toilets or even in pornography - a constant affirmation that something is really wrong with you. Perhaps in the past, you've been reminded by other bullying males of your small penis size or partners from the past or present. Maybe you have gone through lots of frustration getting a condom that fits well. Part or all of this gradually increases your low self-esteem and lack of confidence. Moreover, the media contributes largely to this by giving a seemingly endless focus on the penis size that continually reinforces the assertion that size counts around you. If you have had sexual experiences and your performance was judged to be inadequate, this only cements the idea that your small penis is to blame, and less self-confidence is inevitable.

✓ **Decreased Sexual Satisfaction**

Apart from the emotional consequences, this problem has other 'physical' effects. Sometimes having a small member can lead to reduced sexual satisfaction in women. There was a study done in 2000 by the University of Texas-Pan America that discovered that out of 50 women that were questioned, up to 45 stated that a fairly thick penis was essential in sexual satisfaction. The study stated that reason behind the significance of girth (thickness) is because women want their vaginal walls filled by a penis (containing a large enough surface area) to reach the sensory nerve receptors efficiently. The study also shows that a thicker penis actually increases the levels of sexual satisfaction and in particular in women. *So... how does the bigger member do it?*

A bigger penis causes the vagina to stretch a little bit, causing it to form some sort of a tube shape. This makes every section of the inner walls reachable, including the so-called 'G-spot'. A woman requires this kind of stimulation in order to reach vaginal orgasms. As I mentioned, the vaginal walls have thousands of sensory nerve endings and the more surface contact is made, the more of these will be stimulated at any given time. A larger penis therefore enables you to rub in more surface area, leading to the stimulation of more nerves at once.

✓ **Issues During Sex**

It's quite logical that having small penis can create a couple of problems during intercourse which can seriously affect you a lot. The act of sex itself can be adversely disturbed and some methods of contraception affected immensely. For instance, a condom that does not fit well can slip off quite easily during sex. This can lead to the spread of sexually transmitted infections (STIs). Similarly, having a thin penis can decrease sexual pleasure in your partner or your level of sexual gratification because the vaginal walls cannot fully grip a penis that is already thin.

I know you probably have experienced many or all the downsides of having a small member and are looking for a solution. But before we get to the solutions, let's first answer one more question; what could possibly cause you to have a small member? We will learn that next.

Small Penis Syndrome: What Causes It?

Lucky for you, there are a number of natural, proven ways that can correct your small penis and enlarge both its girth and length. Before I delve into these enlargement techniques, let me explain briefly the cause of the small penis in the first place.

The main cause of small penis size is simply genetics. In other words, you just inherited your penis size from your parents even though there are factors in your environment and diet that can bring an impact in the final outcome as well.

See your DNA as a blueprint in which your penis' size 'specs' are printed. During the critical stages of growth in your life, your body including your penis grew to the specs encoded in your DNA and once the goal, which is indicated by your DNA blueprint was attained, the growth stopped.

Definitely, your body used a lot of energy and resources such as proteins and sugars to grow the new tissue, and obviously, these resources originated from the food you consumed. This is where the diet comes in and thus, it has an impact. You cannot build a skyscraper without enough bricks now can you? However, if the blueprint calls/demands for a two-story building, it is very difficult to convince your body to add extra floors simply by availing more bricks!

What's more, another research has found that there is a correlation between a chemical compound known as Phthalates that is used in many consumer products, paints, pesticides and also PVC pipes with small penis; more specifically, mono 2-ethylhexyl phthalate (MEHP) a component of this compound has been isolated. What's unbelievable is that this chemical is found in poultry- a fact that has led many scientists to believing (after proving) that eating chicken by pregnant mothers can cause small penis in their baby boys. Perhaps chicken is not good for pregnant mothers because it has also been associated with increased odds in cesarean section, male breast growth, attention deficit, diminished child intelligence and hyperactivity disorder symptoms.

But how about the micropenis?

The micropenis in particular is caused by the failure of the male baby's penis from lengthening after the first trimester of pregnancy. It is thought that inadequate testosterone (a male sex hormone) levels in the second and third pregnancy trimesters are caused by its inadequate production during these stages or when the unborn child is not responding well to the amount produced.

According to a research done in Japan, which was also published in the journal of clinical endocrinology and metabolism, genetic mutations of a gene referred to as SRD5A2 can lead to your having a micropenis.

Moreover, the researchers discovered that there are some environmental factors, which could trigger a genetic condition that makes boys more predisposed to developing a micropenis. Such environmental conditions may include the consumption of MEHP (check above) and other chemicals such as pesticides.

The Change You Need

Now you know that most causes of small penis syndrome are quite difficult to avoid (or not avoidable at all). However, with the development in knowledge and in particular, the growth in human understanding of the entire functioning of the human body, people like me have managed to grab and combine accurate information disseminated by scientists out there to provide solutions to problems related to the functioning of the penis among other parts, which have caused headaches and mental distress to many people. The knowledge concerning penile enlargement is backed by the molecular and clinical comprehension of the erectile function that keeps gaining ground every day. Moreover, advances in gene discovery have assisted in working knowledge of smooth relaxation and contraction muscle pathways that has enabled us greatly to gather the necessary facts to come up with conclusive information on PE. Intensive research has brought about numerous advances, which we continue to take advantage of every time.

Therefore, based on various findings, I can comfortably tell you that there are particular parts of your penis, which we can alter in order to increase your penis' length and girth. These areas include:

- ✓ The corpora cavernosa; since the cavernous smooth musculature and the smooth arteriolar-based smooth muscles do play a key role in the erectile process and general enlarging of your penis.

- ✓ The other section is the corpus spongiosum, which is also involved in multiple processes that lead to penile enlargement to a certain level though.

Let's hop into the natural methods (exercises), which will assist us achieve this goal of altering critical parts of your penis to increase your penis' length and girth and make your dreams come true.

The Penis Enlargement Exercises

Girth is the distance measured around an object. I will discuss the natural ways through which you can increase your penis girth and length naturally by using the safest exercises, which are tested and proven to actually work and give excellent results.

Note: Natural is better dive

You have to understand that enlarging your penis is a long term commitment. Regardless of what the scammers out there are saying, popping some penis enlargement pills will do nothing more that give you a temporary increase in the hang, and the story is just the same when you use an ointment, cream or apply a patch.

Going natural provides you a permanent solution and you don't experience side effects, which are not uncommon in numerous artificial methods such as the ones I mentioned above, or even getting a hormonal boost.

The penis exercises, which are specifically created to increase the girth alone includes first one: Jelqing, which has various levels as you will notice as we continue.

Jelqing

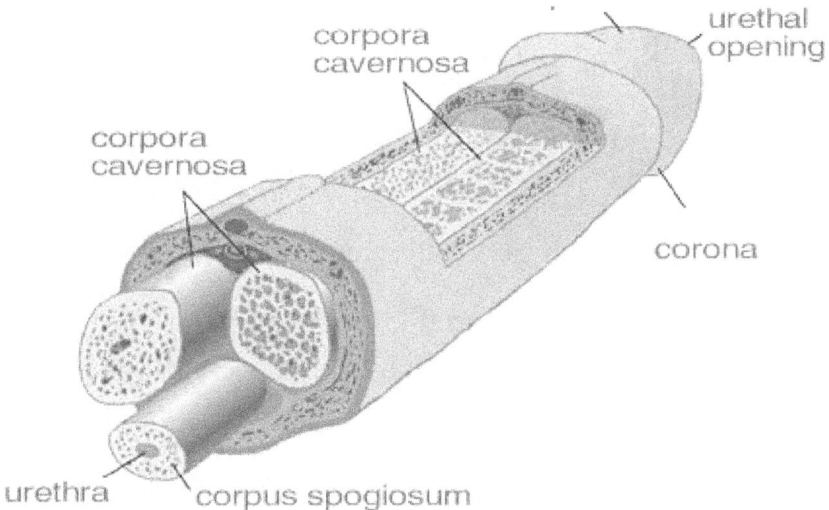

This exercise is one of the best natural girth increasing exercises. The incessant jelq squeezing makes more blood enter the corpora cavernosa (check above) and thus the cell walls expand and stretch in order to get more quantities of blood flowing into the penis, which ultimately increases the girth and length.

Jelqing is actually an ancient technique that was used to increase weight, thickness and density for a proportionately puffed-up member. It is important because as it increases blood flow into the penis, it forces the spaces within to accommodate more blood. Due to this, jelqing is generally considered to be a girth exercise that we cannot afford to leave out. However, there are some people who claim that it does increase the length as well.

Note: The different jeqing exercises are based on this principle but there are some minor variations among them, which you'll notice as you read on.

How To Perform The Exercise

Method 1 (Warming up)

What you need
A washcloth
Warm water

1. Start by massaging your penis until you get a partial erection (semi-tumescent).

2. Get the wash cloth and soak it in the warm water

3. Shawl the cloth around your penis for three minutes (making sure to soak it over and over again in the warm water, as the warmth diminishes)

4. Repeat the warm wrap above for extra three minutes

Method 2

The other option of doing this exercise entails massaging and stroking your semi-tumescent penis in a warm bath.
During the initial weeks of using your thumb and forefinger to create an 'O' or 'okay sign', you have to grip your penis firmly at the base to 'milk' your penis in order to drive blood to the tip. Every motion you make from the base to the tip should take 3 seconds.
What you need
A lubricant like baby oil

1. Start by ensuring your penis is semi erect by massaging it for a short while.

2. Pour a bit of lubricant such as baby oil on your hands and penis.

3. Use your forefinger and thumb of one of your hands and make an 'okay' sign around the base of your penis and give it a firm grip.

4. Next, begin a milking motion in the direction of the tip of your penis

5. When the hand you are using to do this reaches the tip/head of your penis, create an 'okay' sign using the hand that is free and begin milking just like you did previously while using your other hand. Note: you do not milk the head of the penis.

6. Just make sure to use both your hands to create a continuous milking act, each one at a time.

Once you've gotten the hang of this exercise, you can head on to the next:

The Advanced Jelqing: Double Handed Jelq

This exercise improves your member by far in terms of size. Jelqing has become very popular nowadays, and many people have discovered several ways of doing it to improve both length and girth of the penis. I can guarantee you therefore that by the end of this program, you'll have reached the size you've always wanted.

1. Begin this exercise by using your right hand and move it up your shaft to cover about an inch.

2. With your left hand, hold the base where your right hand was (before it moved up) in order to trap the blood inside.

3. Let your right hand jelq up to the section beneath the head. At this moment, you should have more blood trapped within. As the right hand loosens the grip and releases, try to have the left hand jelq up to that same spot beneath the head, but this time, the right hand holding firmly the base.

4. Try maintaining this lengthening cycle while you maintain your hard on at about 95 percent.

The Girth-Specific Jelq

Double handed girth bend
This exercise is solely meant to increase the girth of your penis.
You need to begin as you did with the previous exercise, where your hand is positioned well at the base and the other just below the head. With a large amount of blood trapped inside already, maintain a firm grip while pushing your hands together for 45-60 seconds, driving blood outward.
Caution: don't forget that you should warm up your penis correctly and sufficiently before starting the process. It should remain 95% erect.
The double-handed girth bend
Grab both ends of your shaft, one hand on each end and start bending your penis frontwards, gently from top to bottom for 45 seconds. To repeat this process, bend it towards the opposite side.
The ultimate (final) girth jelq
Start the same way you did with the double handed girth jelq but this time, trying to bring your hands closer together until they are almost touching, as you move along the shaft for 45 seconds.

Focus on the exact areas on the shaft where you want more expansions. In order to get more gains at the base, allow your base hand to stay longer or keep the upper hand solid. You need to vary the exercise depending on the places where you want more gains in girth.

Just like the previous exercise, you need to warm up before doing this exercise and keep your erection at 95%.

Erect Squeeze Exercise

This is another important exercise that naturally increases your penis girth; you want your penis to be thicker so you have to do this too. You should not get comfortable with jeqing alone.

Also known as ULI, the Erect Squeeze Exercise is most effective for expanding the upper shaft and the glans. This exercise also makes the blood in the lower area of the erect penis flow well into the glans and upper shaft.

It is quite a straightforward exercise as it is effective. For this exercise, the ideal erection level is between 50% -90%.

How to perform this exercise

1. Use your left hand to hold the base of your shaft. Let your right hand remain gripping the shaft just behind the head.

2. With your both hands, squeeze and hold for about thirty seconds, then release.

3. Ensure to take a break (between 5-10 seconds) between each repetition.

Note: It is possible to perform this exercise being fully erect. But since this means there will be less buildup of pressure which is very essential, it is less effective.

4. In order to make the ULI more effective, you can try to condense your PC muscles as you perform the squeeze; it will definitely enhance the blood pressure in your penis.

Note: the pubococcygeus muscle (PC) is a hammock-like muscle that is also found in females, which expands from the pubic bone to the tail bone (coccyx), establishing the floor of the pelvic cavity and holding/supporting the pelvic organs. This muscle can also be described as the pelvic floor muscle because it supports your bowel, bladder and uterus (for women). This is the muscle that can cut your urine flow since it's the one you use to stop the flow. So, if you want to find these muscles, just try to cut your urine flow when you're in the process; that muscle you feel down there is the PC muscle. Premature ejaculation and having problems in holding urine is mostly associated with weak PC muscles.

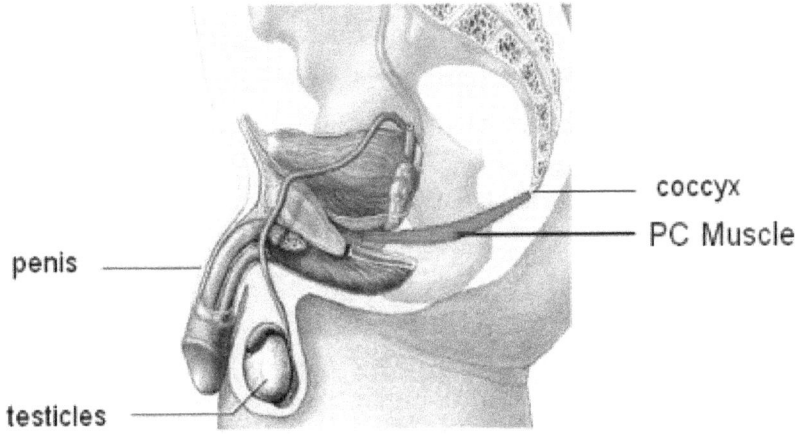

Take care

Note about the risk of injury part: Most of the girth exercises can be quite risky for you if you are new to this. Therefore, take care; if at any point you feel pain while performing the exercises, go slow or even stop and start over some other time, instead of trying to battle with pain, which can lead to damage in the circulatory system of your penis.

Stretching

Right now, we want to generate some tension in the erectile tissues in order to get longer penis ligaments, which will help increase its overall length. Just imagine an impeccable girth and perfect length; what else could possibly beat this combination? So, this one is just as important.

We'll do this by stretching the skin of your penis while erect. This process will generally improve the elasticity of the skin and enlarge the spaces within the corpora cavernosa, an important penis chamber (check the picture above). When these spaces expand, the result is an enlarged penis mass.

How To Perform This Exercise

You need to do four sets of this exercise every day, making sure to warm your penis well each time.

1. Find somewhere to sit: along the edge of your sofa or bed is ideal. Wrap your penis with your index finger and thumb then pull your penis out frontwards for 35 seconds. Apply a gentle, firm grip and start stroking it from the base all the way to the head, while stretching as much skin as you possibly can.

2. Release your penis for 35 seconds.

3. Put it up one more time, directly in front for 35 seconds

4. Next, pull your penis gently towards the left for 35 seconds. Repeat this stretch but towards the right this time for 35 seconds.

5. Start moving the penis in a circular manner for 35 seconds.

After completing these steps, release your penis so that you allow blood to flow normally. If you feel the urge to ejaculate don't hold back, go ahead. However, you need to practice extra caution when performing this exercise because doing it wrongly can cause pain that can cause hurt or serious complications. If you don't feel any pain at all, know that you are most probably doing the right thing because you're not supposed to feel any pain. To be sure, reread the instructions and go slowly any moment you feel pain.

Once you get used to this exercise, you can move on to the next one:

Advanced Stretching

Wrist stretching

In this form of stretching, you apply some pressure on the mid-section of your penis to stretch your ligaments further.

Note: to do this, you have to have trained with jelqing and the basic stretching.

Just like the basic stretch, grip your penis just beneath the head and stretch it frontwards, then left to right, up and down. The pressure added will come from your free hand wrist that will be pressing down to the middle of the shaft as you stretch it. As you stretch to the left side, apply wrist pressure on the left side of the shaft but when stretching upwards, direct the pressure towards the other side and so on.

Big-seated stretch

This one is a non-stop stretch that is supposed to take 10 minutes for each stretch exercise. It requires more privacy therefore.

You only require sitting with one leg raised up and your hand beneath. Then reach out to hold/grip right below the head and then pull with full force, without letting go for ten minutes. Repeat this process with your other hand and opposite leg.

The Big Squeeze

This exercise is more like a stretch and it requires you to take particular steps of squeezing your penis.

You only need to lay your penis on a table and then use both of your hands (one on top of the other) to squeeze down on the penis (covering it with your palm). Make sure to carefully press it with all of your weight. Keep doing this for about 45 seconds.

Warming Down

After an exercise, you need to allow your penis to recover by rebuilding the worn out cell tissues quicker. You therefore have to make sure you warm down at the end of each exercise using a hot towel. Once you cover your penis with the hot towel, massage it gently for one minute. Run your middle fingers and forefingers along the shaft and base. You need to be gentle because your penis will definitely be tender after the exercises. When you finish massaging, apply the heat once more to stimulate the parts in your penis to function well.

The Penis Exercises Schedule

If you feel you need a schedule to follow, I will now give one to you. The exercises remain the same but since this is a schedule, you will notice that some of the intervals have changed (compared to those in the exercises above). You may not be able to see the improvements immediately but once enough nutrients are absorbed and a couple of weeks into exercising, you definitely will. You have to get prepared for better erections too but real gains will come after the first ten weeks. When you combine the penis enlargement exercises with a proper diet, you are well on your path to a larger penis and better performance in bed.

Between the 1ˢᵗ and 3ʳᵈ week, use 15-twenty minutes each day to perform the basic jelqing and basic stretching.

1. Start by preparing the penis with a gentle massage and warm piece of cloth for 2-3 minutes. Next, do the standard stretching with each stretch (left, right, up, down) taking 30 seconds. Make sure to keep your penis flaccid here to avoid hurting yourself.

2. Now, try to flex your PC muscles (as you would do when holding your urine) and hold as long as you possibly can then relax. After twenty minutes, rest shortly and then use a warm towel to wrap your penis to help it rest before repeating the exercise.

3. Do a basic jelq for 10 minutes and then perform the warm down. Do it for 5 days then rest for 2 days and see if you'll start noticing an improved erection. Do a double handed jelq for 10 minutes on the third week.

Between the 4ᵗʰ and 5ᵗʰ week, perform these exercises for 15-20 minutes each day.

1. Start with the basic stretching using your two hands, the stroking should last 3-5 seconds. Make sure to keep the penis flaccid.

2. Next, do the standard jelqing for 5 minutes and make sure to alternate your hands in the process.

3. Do the wrist stretch for 5 minutes.

4. For two minutes, do the big squeeze.

Between the 6th and 8th week, do the following for 20-30 minutes each day.

This is the last transitional phase to the end of the cycle and by this time, your body should be feeling better by this time. So far, you don't need to do anything further but based on your daily activities, you can look for means to have your exercises split, for instance, have some in the morning and others in the evening so that you prepare your penis effectively for the advanced exercises.

Over time, your penis will become ready for more; therefore, you can start doing the advanced jelqs and stretches but save the double-handed girth bend and ultimate girth for later. You can do them for half an hour a day.

Slowly, you'll feel when your penis and body in general is ready for the more advanced exercises. At this point, you can perform all the exercises but focusing on those which you'll have noticed your body responding best to. Ensure you vary your routines for maximum results.

During the 8th week, take 15 minutes on each intense workout

At this point, you are much more comfortable performing the routines and since you are ready to create your own, add more variations but keeping in mind the exercises that work best for you.

The Penis Enlargement Food Advice

So, you have begun exercising. Good. That will make your member larger than it is over time. What you need now is boost your efforts to get your penis 'there' quicker and easier, while keeping your entire body healthy too. There are particular foods you need to start taking in order to achieve that. The best thing about it is that the foods I'll mention are found almost everywhere; supermarkets, small and large fruit and meat outlets and several vendor-stalls – you cannot say that you can't access any of these foods.

What To Eat

Note: most of these foods are listed because they either improve blood circulation or heal penile tissues, which we need right now -the amount of these foods you'll eat will be an issue of personal preference.

1. **Watermelon**

Watermelon has an essential amino acid known as citrulline that is converted in the body to another amino acid known as arginine, which is very penis friendly. Arginine therefore relaxes your blood vessels, producing an effect similar to that of Viagra. This substance also improves your circulatory system (essential in the P.E) and immune system to keep your body healthy and disease to exercise better.

2. **Liver**

Liver contains natural properties that make it a major vasodilator (a substance that widens the arteries) in order to allow more blood to flow throughout the body. As you well know, penis enlargement requires widening of blood vessels and improved blood flow.

3. Fish

I recommend you go for Tuna or Salmon because apart from the essential omega three fatty acids you need to have good health in general, you need low calories for better cardiovascular health. This will enable more blood to pump throughout the body to give you a bigger erection.

4. Oysters/spinach

For a very long time, oysters have been used to increase libido and penis size. If you look closely on the labels of male enhancement and enlargement supplements, you'll not miss zinc. Oysters and spinach are loaded with this element, which is important in penile enlargement. When you are exercising, you damage tissues. In order to heal these tissues and thus increase the size of your penis, you need zinc.

5. Yellow bell pepper

Famous for its high Vitamin C levels, this pepper is very important in growing body cells, repair of tissues (crucial in your exercise schedule) and sustaining a healthy sexual function. All these benefits come from its high vitamin C content. With a yellow bell pepper of average size, you can get a whopping 569% of your day to day vitamin C value.

What To Avoid

Alcohol

Alcohol reduces and affects the production of testosterone. This is a very important hormone in the growth of your penis. In as much as you may be working hard to enlarge your penis, alcohol can easily frustrate your efforts because reduction in testosterone has been proven to be a leading cause of penis shrinking.

Smoking

Smoking affects the penis the exact same way it does the heart. The smoke destroys the blood vessels and inhibits the normal flow of blood. Moreover, smoking can actually reduce the size of your penis since it restricts the blood flowing into the chambers within your penis - the penis is among the first and quickest areas in the body to suffer from clogged arteries.

High fats (especially saturated fats)

You have to reduce or eliminate your intake of high fat diets because they raise the level of blood cholesterol in your body, something which (over time) makes your arteries grow very thin. The pudendal arteries that carry blood to your penis are not spared either. Examples of foods containing high saturated fats include: cheese, heavy cream, butter, processed meat such as bacon and Italian salami.

High doses (excessive) dietary fiber

I know this is quite a surprise for you. Fiber definitely is a good thing because it lowers the levels of cholesterol in your body and enhances satiety after meals besides balancing blood glucose levels really well in your body.

The problem with too much fiber is that in most cases, it reduces the levels of testosterone in your body. You need to be moderate in your fiber consumption therefore.

Soy

This food has been shown to reduce testosterone in a very important study done and published by the Society for Endocrinology. If you want high protein, you don't have to go for soy since there are many other options such as fish.

Conclusion

As you have noted, enlarging your penis naturally is possible after all. Needless to say, the exercises I have explained above are the best you can ever get in pursuit for the ideal penis that every man wants.

Just make sure not to forget my advice about the foods; it will help you especially throughout your exercising period.

Thank you again for downloading this book!
I hope this book was able to help you to understand how to increase the girth and length of your penis naturally without any equipment and possible side effects.
The next step is to implement what you have learnt.

Finally, if you enjoyed this book, would you be kind enough to leave a review for this book on Amazon?

Click here to leave a review for this book on Amazon!

Thank you and good luck!